MACRO DIET COOKBOOK
FOR

BEGINNERS 2024

An All-Inclusive Strategy for Health, Wellness, and Mindfulness

Garry N. Mullet

Table of Content

INTRODUCTION
Choosing Macronutrient Ratios
Consider the following while designing your dietary plan
Ratio Adjustment for Various Goals
Tools and ingredients required
Macro Cooking Kitchen Equipment
Macro-Friendly Ingredients You Must Have
Meal Planning Fundamentals

CHAPTER 1
Breakfast Ideas
Omelet with Protein:
Parfait with Greek Yogurt
Smoothie Bowl with Protein:
4. Avocado Toast with Whole Grain
Scrambled Egg Whites with Veggies

CHAPTER 2
Lunch Suggestions
Quinoa Bowl with Grilled Chicken:
Salad with Shrimp and Avocado
Wrap with turkey and hummus
Salad with lentils and chickpeas
Bowl of Sweet Potatoes with Black Beans

CHAPTER 3
Dinner Favorites

Salmon Baked with Quinoa and Asparagus
Stir-fry with Turkey and Vegetables
Bell Pepper Stuffed with Quinoa and Black Beans
Skewers of chicken and vegetables with cauliflower rice
Curry with Lentils and Vegetables

CHAPTER 4
Snacks and Side Dishes
Guacamole with Carrot Sticks
Greek Yogurt and Berry Parfait
Platter of Hummus and Veggies
Cups of Cottage Cheese and Pineapple
Baked Sweet Potato Fries
Protein-Packed Deviled Eggs
Nuts and Seeds Trail Mix

CHAPTER 5
Sweet Treats
Chocolate Protein Smoothie
Greek Yogurt Parfait with Berries and Granola
Energy Bites with Banana and Peanut Butter
Mixed Berry Chia Seed Pudding
Apple Baked with Cinnamon and Walnuts
Protein Ice Cream with Mixed Berries
Oatmeal Banana Cookies

CHAPTER 6
Eating Out While Following a Macro Diet
CHAPTER 7

Troubleshooting and guidance for a successful journey through the macro diet

Concerns Regarding Deficiencies in Nutrients

CHAPTER 8

Sample Meal Plans for a Balanced Macro Diet

Meal Plan 1

Basics in Balance

Plant-Based Delights

Meal Plan 2

Meal Plan 3

High-Impact Day

Meal Plan 4

Simple and Quick Options

Mediterranean-Inspired Meal Plan 5 Delights

Meal Plan 6

Vegetarian Options

Meal Plan 7

Low-Carb Alternatives

Meal Plan 8

Remixed Comfort Food

Meal Plan 9

Easy and Healthy

Meal Plan 10

Protein-Rich Options

CHAPTER 9

Fitness and Macros: A Complete Overview

CHAPTER 10

CONCLUSION

INTRODUCTION

Welcome to the exciting world of macro dieting, where nutrition and precision combine to change the way you eat and fuel your body. This cookbook is your entire guide to mastering the art of macronutrients, whether you're a fitness expert trying to improve your diet or someone just starting on their health journey.

Macronutrients Explained

The macro diet is built around the careful study of macronutrients—proteins, carbs, and fats. Each of these is essential for supporting your body's processes and accomplishing your health and fitness objectives. Proteins help in muscle repair and growth, carbs offer energy, and fats help with hormonal balance and overall health. By learning to balance these macronutrients, you acquire the ability to adjust your diet to your specific needs.

Macro Diet Advantages for Beginners

Beginning a macro diet journey has numerous advantages, especially for people who are unfamiliar with the notion. In contrast to restrictive diets that focus simply on calorie reduction, macro dieting focuses on the quality and balance of your food intake. This method not only promotes long-term weight management but also a healthier connection with food. We hope that this cookbook will help to simplify the complexities of macro dieting, making it more approachable and fun for newcomers.

Starting with Macro Tracking

Tracking your daily intake is one of the pillars of a successful macro diet. Don't worry; it's easier than it sounds. We'll walk you through the process of calculating your personal macronutrient requirements based on parameters like age, weight, exercise level, and goals. With this knowledge, you'll be able to determine reasonable macronutrient ratios that correspond with your goals, whether they're to lose a few pounds, grow muscle, or simply live a healthy lifestyle.

As you go through the pages of this cookbook, you'll discover not only delicious and gratifying meals, but also the skills you need to maximize your nutrition. We'll go over basic kitchen equipment and must-have supplies to make your culinary adventure as easy as it is nutritious.

Meal Planning Fundamentals

Efficient meal planning is the foundation of macro dieting success. In this part, we'll reveal the secrets of weekly meal prep, presenting ideas to help you save time in the kitchen and ensure a week of balanced, delicious meals. Learn how to prepare meals that not only meet your macronutrient requirements, but also your taste preferences and lifestyle.

Choosing Macronutrient Ratios

Understanding the optimal macronutrient ratios for your objectives is critical. Whether you want to lose weight, add muscle, or keep your present shape, we'll walk you through the process of altering your macronutrient ratios. This individualized approach ensures that your nutrition plan is tailored to your specific trip.

Tools and ingredients required

Stock up on macro-friendly ingredients and equip your kitchen with the required gear. We'll present a thorough list of items to make your cooking experience fun and efficient, ranging from measuring cups and scales to nutrient-dense ingredients that improve your meals.

Rest assured that variety and flavor will not be sacrificed as you embark on this macro diet adventure. We've compiled a collection of dishes for breakfast, lunch, dinner, snacks, and even sweet desserts, all with a focus on balance and flavor. Discover protein-packed breakfasts, macro-friendly salads, one-pan marvels, and guilt-free treats that rethink the concept of healthy eating.

We'll address frequent issues and provide troubleshooting advice along the way to keep you on track. We've got you covered on everything from browsing restaurant menus to changing your macros based on progress. This cookbook is more than simply a recipe compilation; it's your go-to guide for mastering the macro lifestyle.

So, whether you're a seasoned chef or a culinary novice, join us in unlocking the potential of macro dieting. Let's begin on a trip that will not only improve your plate but also change your perspective on nutrition. Cheers to a happier, healthier you!

Choosing Macronutrient Ratios

Understanding and fine-tuning your macronutrient ratios is like holding the key to a personalized and effective nutrition plan in the world of macro dieting. This section will serve as your guide, helping you through the process of calculating and modifying your macronutrient ratios based on your specific goals, whether they are weight loss, muscle gain, or maintaining a healthy lifestyle.

Personal Macronutrient Needs Calculation

It's critical to establish your baseline before delving into the specifics of macronutrient ratios. Age, weight, gender, exercise level, and overall fitness goals all have an impact on your specific macronutrient requirements. This cookbook gives simple ways to calculate your daily caloric requirements and then determine the macronutrient proportion that best matches your goals.

Consider the following while designing your dietary plan

Weight and Body Composition

The amount of protein you require, a critical macronutrient for muscle maintenance, is frequently determined by your body weight. Understanding your body composition aids in setting realistic protein intake goals.

Activity Level

Those who lead an active lifestyle may require greater carbohydrate consumption to meet their energy requirements, while fat intake may need to be adjusted based on overall caloric requirements.

Goals

Determining your goals, whether they are weight loss, muscle gain, or weight maintenance, has a direct impact on your macronutrient ratios. A larger protein intake, for example, may be prioritized for muscle building, but a managed calorie deficit may be required for weight loss.

Ratio Adjustment for Various Goals

Once you've determined your baseline macronutrient requirements, you can fine-tune the ratios based on your unique goals.

Weight Loss

If your primary goal is to lose weight, a moderate calorie deficit is usually used. This entails modifying your macronutrient ratios to guarantee enough protein consumption to maintain lean muscle mass, a modest quantity of healthy fats, and controlled carbohydrates to achieve a calorie deficit.

Muscle Gain

A little calorie excess is often recommended for people looking to gain muscle. This entails boosting your protein consumption to stimulate muscle building, changing your carbohydrate intake to give energy for workouts, and including healthy fats to improve your general well-being.

If you want to keep your present weight and body composition, your macronutrient ratios will be modified to match your calorie needs. This frequently entails a well-balanced combination of proteins, carbs, and fats to support general health and energy needs.

Understanding the importance of each macronutrient in reaching your objectives is critical. Proteins, which are essential for muscle repair and growth, should be prioritized throughout muscular growth phases. Carbohydrates, the body's primary source of energy, are essential for fueling workouts and maintaining an active lifestyle. Fats, which are sometimes misinterpreted, are necessary for hormone production, cognitive function, and overall health.

This portion of the cookbook is intended to demystify the process of establishing and modifying macronutrient ratios, making it approachable and actionable for beginners. We empower you to navigate the delicate mix of proteins, carbs, and fats to fulfill your particular health and fitness goals by giving clear recommendations and practical tips.

As you go through the pages, you'll discover not just theoretical information on macronutrient ratios, but also practical applications. Sample meal plans adapted to different goals, as well as insights into altering ratios based on your progress, ensure that you're establishing a sustainable and personalized approach to nutrition rather than just following a diet.

So, whether you're trying to lose weight, grow muscle, or simply live a healthy lifestyle, this section will teach you how to determine macronutrient ratios that will help you achieve your goals. Welcome to a life-changing experience in which precision meets nutrition and your plate becomes a painting for reaching your health and fitness goals.

Tools and ingredients required

As you begin your macro diet adventure, stocking up on vital foods and equipping your kitchen with the necessary tools is the first step in creating nutritious, balanced, and delicious meals. This section of the cookbook will walk you through the tools and ingredients that will not only speed your cooking process but also ensure that your culinary creations are in sync with your macronutrient goals.

Macro Cooking Kitchen Equipment

In the realm of macro dieting, a well-equipped kitchen is your secret weapon. Here's a list of the essential items you'll need to make your cooking experience both efficient and enjoyable:

Food Scale:

Precision is essential in macro dieting, and a dependable food scale is your best ally for correct portioning and ingredient tracking.

Measuring Cups and Spoons:

These essential tools are essential for correctly measuring liquids, grains, and other components to keep your macronutrient ratios balanced.

Quality Knife Set:

A sharp, high-quality knife set is essential for quick meal prep, allowing you to easily slice and dice your items.

Nonstick Cookware:

Invest in nonstick pans and pots to reduce the need for extra cooking oils, supporting a healthier approach to meal preparation.

Blender or Food Processor:

These flexible equipment are ideal for making smoothies, sauces, and homemade dressings, as they allow you to regulate the components and keep them within your macronutrient targets.

Baking Sheets and Pans:

Having quality baking sheets and pans is essential for those delectable macro-friendly desserts and one-pan dinners.

7. Meal Prep Containers:

Plan ahead of time and portion your foods into meal prep containers. This not only saves you time, but it also keeps you on track with your dietary goals.

Macro-Friendly Ingredients You Must Have

Let's get started with the cupboard and refrigerator basics that will serve as the foundation of your macro diet adventure. These components are not only nutrient-dense, but they are also adaptable, allowing you to make a wide range of meals without losing flavor.

1. Proteins that are low in fat:

• Chicken Thighs

• Turkey's

• Tender Beef

• Seafood (Salmon, Cod, Tilapia)

• Eggs

• Yogurt from Greece

• Tofu

• Legumes

2. complex Carbohydrates:

• Quinoa.

• Basmati rice

• Baked Sweet Potatoes

• Oats

• Pasta with Whole Grain

• Grain barley

• Farro

3. Fats that are good for you:

• Avocado

• Extra Virgin Olive Oil

• Nuts (walnuts, almonds)

• Seeds (Chia, Flaxseeds)

• Nut jars of butter (such as peanut butter and almond butter)

4. Vegetables:

- Brussel sprouts

- Lettuce

- Kale

- Red bell peppers

- Cucumber

- Broccoli Sprouts

- Cauliflower is a vegetable.

5. Fruits:

- Berries (strawberries, blueberries, raspberries)

- Apple

- Banana

- Citrus fruits

- Mango

- The pineapple

6. Dairy or Dairy Substitutes:

• Low-Fat Cheddar

• Almond, Soy, or Skim Milk

• Cottage Cheddar

• Yogurt from Greece

7. Spices and herbs:

• Herbs (basil, cilantro, and parsley)

• Fresh garlic

• Garlic

• Curcuma

• Cumin

• Chilean paprika

• Cardamom

Having these components on hand guarantees that your meals are not just high in macronutrients but also high in flavor. Because of their adaptability, these mainstays allow you to experiment with different combinations, keeping your macro diet interesting and sustainable.

As you work your way through the recipes in this book, you'll notice that the combination of the correct equipment and high-quality ingredients sets the setting for culinary success. This section empowers you to transform your kitchen into a refuge for macro-friendly creations, from exact measures to imaginative food preparations. So gather your supplies, stock your cupboard, and prepare to begin on a wonderful and nutritious macro diet adventure!

Meal Planning Fundamentals

In the world of macro dieting, meal preparation is critical to success. It is more than just preparing meals; it is a deliberate approach to ensuring that your nutrition is in line with your goals. In this section, we'll go over the basics of meal planning, giving you the tools you need to make informed decisions, streamline your cooking process, and set yourself up for long-term success.

1. Knowing Your Macronutrient Goals:

Before you begin planning your meals, you must understand your macronutrient targets. These goals will serve as the foundation for your meal planning efforts, directing the distribution of proteins, carbs, and fats in each meal. To define your daily targets, apply what you learned in the preceding section on setting macronutrient ratios.

2. Weekly Meal Preparation Techniques:

When it comes to meal planning, efficiency is everything, and weekly meal prep is your hidden weapon. Consider setting out a day each week to plan, shop for, and cook your meals. Here's a step-by-step method to weekly meal prep success:

• Menu Planning:

Begin by sketching out your weekly menu. Breakfast, lunch, supper, and any snacks are all included. A well-thought-out plan not only avoids decision fatigue but also guarantees that you have all of the necessary elements on hand.

• Make a Shopping List:

Create a thorough shopping list based on your meal. This reduces the possibility of impulse purchases and ensures you have everything you need to carry out your meal plan.

• Batch Cooking:

Look for meals that can be prepared in bulk and stored for several days. One-pot meals, casseroles, and slow-cooker dishes are wonderful options for batch cooking.

• Portion Control:

Once your meals are prepared, portion them into containers depending on your macronutrient goals. This not only helps you track your intake but also prevents you from deviating from your plan.

• Variety and Flexibility:

While planning is essential, leave room for improvisation. Include a variety of recipes to keep your dinners interesting, and don't be afraid to make changes based on your preferences and time constraints.

3. Creating Macro-Balanced Meals:

Effective meal planning is all about balancing macronutrients throughout each meal. Consider the following guidelines while preparing well-rounded, macro-friendly meals:

• Protein First:

Base every meal on a lean protein source. Protein, whether it's chicken, tofu, or lentils, is important for muscle maintenance and controlling hunger.

• Smart carbs:

Include complex carbs such as whole grains, sweet potatoes, and quinoa in your diet to offer energy throughout the day.

- **Healthy Fats:**

Include sources of healthy fats, such as avocados, almonds, or olive oil, in your diet to improve overall health and flavor.

- **Colorful Vegetables:**

Pile your plate high with colorful vegetables. They not only provide necessary vitamins and minerals, but they also enhance the visual appearance of your cuisine.

4. Changing for Different Days:

Recognize that your dietary requirements may change from day to day depending on your activity level, workouts, or social activities. Consider changing your macronutrient distribution and portion levels. On more active days, you may have more carbohydrates to fuel your exercises, but rest days may require a slightly different distribution.

5. Convenience and portability:

Include meals that are simple to transport, especially if you lead a hectic schedule. Invest in portable containers and prepare snacks or meals for on-the-go consumption. This guarantees that you keep on track with your nutrition even if you have a busy schedule.

6. Variety and flavor:

Maintaining an engaging and varied menu is critical for long-term macro diet adherence. To keep your taste buds active, try new herbs, spices, and cooking techniques. A variety of cuisine not only increases overall enjoyment but also guarantees you get a wide range of nutrients.

You can transform your kitchen into a hub of purposeful nourishment by mastering the art of meal planning. The tactics presented in this part empower you to take charge of your food, transforming macro dieting into a sustainable and pleasurable lifestyle rather than just a routine. Use these meal planning essentials as your foundation as you work your way through the cookbook, paving the road for a successful and happy macro diet journey.

CHAPTER 1

Breakfast Ideas

Start your day off properly with these nutrient-dense breakfast recipes that not only taste fantastic but also fit into your macro diet goals. Each recipe is carefully prepared with a balanced combination of proteins, carbs, and healthy fats to jumpstart your metabolism and deliver continuous energy throughout the morning.

Omelet with Protein:

Ingredients:

• three huge eggs

• 1/4 cup chopped (any color) bell peppers

• 1/4 cup chopped tomatoes

• 1/4 cup chopped onions

• 1/4 cup low-fat shredded cheese

• Season with salt and pepper to taste

• 1 tablespoon olive oil for cooking

Instructions:

1. Whisk the eggs in a mixing dish and season with salt and pepper.

2. In a nonstick skillet over medium heat, heat the olive oil.

3. Cook until the bell peppers, tomatoes, and onions are softened.

4. Pour the whisked eggs evenly over the vegetables.

5. On one half of the omelet, sprinkle it with shredded cheese.

6. Fold the omelet in half when the edges begin to set.

7. Cook until the cheese melts and the eggs are done.

Approximate nutritional value:

- 350 calories

- 25g protein

- 10g Carbohydrates

- Fat: 22g

Parfait with Greek Yogurt

Ingredients:

- 1 cup plain nonfat Greek yogurt

- 1/2 cup berry mixture (strawberries, blueberries, raspberries)

- 1/4 cup granola (low-sugar preferred)

- 1 tablespoon honey for drizzling

Instructions:

1. Layer half of the Greek yogurt in a glass or bowl.

2. Half of the mixed berries should be placed on top of the yogurt layer.

3. Half of the granola should be sprinkled over the berries.

4. Layer the remaining yogurt, berries, and granola over top.

5. To add sweetness, drizzle honey on top.

Approximate nutritional value:

- 300 calories

- 20g protein

- 40g carbohydrates

- Fat: 5g

Smoothie Bowl with Protein:

Ingredients:

- 1 sprinkling of vanilla protein powder

- 1 banana, frozen

- 1/2 cup almond milk, unsweetened

- 1 tablespoon almond butter

- Serve with sliced strawberries, chia seeds, and granola.

Instructions:

1. Combine protein powder, frozen banana, almond milk, and almond butter in a blender.

2. Ensure that the mixture is blended until it reaches a velvety consistency.

3. Fill a bowl halfway with the smoothie.

4. Served with sliced strawberries, chia seeds, and granola on top.

Approximate nutritional value:

• 400 calories

• 30g protein

• 40g carbohydrates

• Fat: 15g

4. Avocado Toast with Whole Grain

Ingredients:

• 2 slices whole-wheat bread

• 1/2 avocado, mashed

• Sliced cherry tomatoes

• Optional red pepper flakes

• Then add salt and pepper

Instructions:

1. Toast the slices of whole-grain bread.

2. Distribute the mashed avocado equally across the toasted bread.

3. Serve with sliced cherry tomatoes on top.

4. Season with salt, pepper, and red pepper flakes, according to your taste.

Approximate nutritional value:

- 300 calories

- 8g protein

- 30g carbohydrates

- Fat: 18g

Scrambled Egg Whites with Veggies

Ingredients:

- 1-quart egg whites

- 1/4 cup bell peppers, chopped

- 1/4 cup chopped spinach

- 1/4 cup halved cherry tomatoes

- 1 tablespoon olive oil for cooking

- Garnish with fresh herbs (such as parsley).

Instructions:

1. Whisk the egg whites in a mixing bowl.

2. Set the olive oil to medium heat in a skillet.

3. Cook until the bell peppers, spinach, and cherry tomatoes are soft.

4. Pour the egg whites over the vegetables.

5. Gently stir until the eggs are fully cooked.

6. Before serving, garnish with fresh herbs.

Approximate nutritional value:

- 150 calories

• 25g protein

• 5g Carbohydrates

• Fat: 3g

These breakfast recipes provide the ideal combination of flavors and nutrition to get your day started. Experiment with these alternatives and feel free to tailor them to your personal tastes and macro goals. Enjoy a substantial and macro-friendly breakfast that will set the tone for the rest of your day.

CHAPTER 2

Lunch Suggestions

Elevate your midday meal with these delicious and nutritious lunch alternatives that are perfectly aligned with your macro diet goals. These dishes are designed to deliver a well-balanced mix of proteins, carbohydrates, and healthy fats, ensuring that your lunch not only tastes good but also fuels your body for the rest of the day.

Quinoa Bowl with Grilled Chicken:

Ingredients:

• 4 ounces sliced grilled chicken breast

• 1/2 cup quinoa, cooked

• 1 cup mixed vegetables

• 1 tablespoon olive oil

• To taste, lemon juice, salt, and pepper

Instructions:

1. Grill the chicken breast until it is fully done, then cut it into strips.

2. Sauté mixed vegetables in olive oil in a skillet until soft.

3. Combine the cooked quinoa and the sautéed vegetables.

4. Serve the quinoa and veggie mixture topped with grilled chicken slices.

5. Season with salt and pepper and drizzle with lemon juice.

Approximate nutritional value:

- 450 calories

- 35g protein

- 35g carbohydrate

- Fat: 18g

Salad with Shrimp and Avocado

Ingredients:

• 6 oz cooked and peeled shrimp

• 1/2 sliced avocado

• 2 cups greens (spinach, arugula, kale)

• Halved cherry tomatoes

• 1 tablespoon olive oil

• To taste, balsamic vinegar, salt, and pepper

Instructions:

1. Combine cooked shrimp, diced avocado, mixed greens, and cherry tomatoes in a mixing dish.

2. Drizzle with balsamic vinegar and olive oil.

3. Toss the salad lightly to distribute the dressing evenly.

4. Then add salt and pepper.

Approximate nutritional value:

- 380 calories

- 25g protein

- 15g carbohydrate

- Fat: 25g

Wrap with turkey and hummus

Ingredients:

- 4 ounces lean turkey slices

- Tortilla (whole-grain or spinach)

- 2 tablespoons hummus

- Greens (lettuce, cucumber, and red onion)

- 1/4 cup carrots, shredded

- 1 tablespoon olive oil

Instructions:

1. Spread the hummus evenly across the tortilla.

2. On one half of the tortilla, layer turkey slices.

3. Top with shredded carrots and mixed greens.

4. Dress with olive oil.

5. Roll the tortilla into a tight coil.

Approximate nutritional value:

• 400 calories

• 30g protein

• 30g carbohydrates

• Fat: 18g

Salad with lentils and chickpeas

Ingredients:

• 1 cup lentils, cooked

- 1/2 cup washed and drained chickpeas

- 1/4 cup crumbled feta cheese

- Halved cherry tomatoes

- Diced cucumber

- Finely sliced red onion

- chopped fresh parsley

- 2 tablespoons olive oil

- Season with pepper, salt, and red wine vinegar to taste.

Instructions:

1. Combine cooked lentils, chickpeas, feta cheese, cherry tomatoes, cucumber, red onion, and fresh parsley in a mixing bowl.

2. Olive oil and red wine vinegar should be drizzled over the dish.

3. Season to taste with salt and pepper.

4. Gently toss the salad until completely incorporated.

Approximate nutritional value:

- 350 calories

- 18g protein

- 40g carbohydrates

- Fat: 15g

Bowl of Sweet Potatoes with Black Beans

Ingredients:

- 1 cup chopped roasted sweet potatoes

- 1/2 cup cooked black beans

- 1/4 cup kernels of corn

- Sliced avocado

- Chopped fresh cilantro

- slices of lime

• • Add salt and chili powder according to personal preference.

Instructions:

1. Sweet potatoes, chopped, roasted till soft.

2. Combine the roasted sweet potatoes, black beans, and corn kernels in a mixing dish.

3. Serve with sliced avocado and fresh cilantro on top.

4. Squeeze lime wedges over the top of the bowl.

5. Season to taste with salt and chili powder.

Approximate nutritional value:

- 420 calories

- 15g protein

- 60g carbohydrates

- Fat: 12g

These lunch options are not only simple to prepare, but also high in nutrients, giving you the energy and sustenance you need to get through the afternoon. Adapt these recipes to your taste preferences and portion sizes while adhering to your macro diet goals.

CHAPTER 3

Dinner Favorites

Finish your day with these delectable and nutritionally balanced dinner recipes that are tailored to your macro diet goals. From one-pan meals to protein-packed feasts, these dishes promise to satisfy your taste senses while also supplying the nutrition your body requires for optimal performance and recuperation.

Salmon Baked with Quinoa and Asparagus

Ingredients:

- 6 ounces salmon filet

- 1/2 cup cooked quinoa

- spears of asparagus

- 1 tablespoon olive oil

- Lemon rind and juice

- Dill, fresh, chopped

- Then add salt and pepper to taste

Instructions:

1. Get the oven up to 375 F (190 C) before you start.

2. Arrange the salmon on a baking sheet, surrounded by asparagus spears.

3. Drizzle olive oil over the fish and asparagus.

4. Season with salt, pepper, and lemon zest if desired.

5. Bake for 15-20 minutes, or until the salmon is thoroughly cooked.

6. Serve with quinoa that has been cooked.

7. Garnish with fresh dill and lemon juice to taste.

Approximate nutritional value:

• 500 calories

• 35g protein

• 30g carbohydrates

• Fat: 25g

Stir-fry with Turkey and Vegetables

Ingredients:

• 8 ounces lean ground turkey

• Florets of broccoli

- Thinly sliced bell peppers

- Green peas

- Julienned carrots

- 2 tablespoons soy sauce

- 1 tablespoon sesame oil

- Minced garlic and ginger

- chopped green onions

- Cooked brown rice

Instructions:

1. Cook ground turkey until browned in a wok or skillet.

2. Sauté for a minute with the minced garlic and ginger.

3. Combine broccoli, bell peppers, snap peas, and carrots in a mixing bowl.

4. Drizzle with sesame oil and soy sauce.

5. Cook until the vegetables are soft.

6. Over-cooked brown rice, serve.

7. Garnish with green onions, sliced.

Approximate nutritional value:

• 450 calories

• 30g protein

• 45g carbohydrate

• Fat: 18g

Bell Pepper Stuffed with Quinoa and Black Beans

Ingredients:

• Assorted colored bell peppers

• 1 cup cooked quinoa

• 1/2 cup cooked black beans

• Corn husks

• Tomatoes, diced

• 1 tablespoon shredded cheddar cheese

- Seasoning for tacos

- Chopped fresh cilantro

- slices of lime

Instructions:

1. Get the oven up to 375 F (190 C) before you start.

2. Remove the seeds from the bell peppers and cut them in half.

3. Combine cooked quinoa, black beans, corn, chopped tomatoes, and taco seasoning in a mixing bowl.

4. Fill each bell pepper half halfway with the quinoa mixture.

5. Shredded cheddar cheese on top.

6. Bake for 20-25 minutes, or until the peppers are soft.

7. Serve with lime wedges and garnished with fresh cilantro.

Approximate nutritional value:

- 380 calories

- 18g protein

- 50g carbohydrates

- Fat: 12g

Skewers of chicken and vegetables with cauliflower rice

Ingredients:

- 8 ounces cubed chicken breast

- Tomatoes, cherry

- Sliced zucchini

- Red onion, peeled and diced

- 1 tablespoon olive oil

- Cumin, paprika, and garlic powder

- Add salt and pepper

- Cooked cauliflower rice

Instructions:

1. Warm up the grill or grill pan.

2. Toss chicken cubes, cherry tomatoes, zucchini, and red onion with olive oil and seasonings in a mixing bowl.

3. Thread onto wooden skewers.

4. Grill the skewers until the chicken is cooked through and the vegetables are slightly browned.

5. Over-cooked cauliflower rice, serve.

Approximate nutritional value:

- 420 calories

- 35g protein

- 20g carbohydrates

- Fat: 20g

Curry with Lentils and Vegetables

Ingredients:

- 1 cup cooked dried lentils

- Vegetables (bell peppers, carrots, and peas)

- 1 can diced tomatoes (14 oz)

- 1 coconut milk can (14 oz)

- 2 tablespoons curry powder

- 1 teaspoon turmeric

- 1 teaspoon cumin

- 1 tablespoon olive oil

- Then add salt and pepper

- Garnish with fresh cilantro

- Cooked brown rice

Instructions:

1. Sauté mixed vegetables in olive oil in a large pot until slightly softened.

2. Cooked lentils, diced tomatoes, coconut milk, and spices are added.

3. Allow flavors to mingle for 15-20 minutes while simmering.

4. Over-cooked brown rice, serve.

5. Garnish with fresh cilantro if desired.

Approximate nutritional value:

• 380 calories

• 20g protein

• 45g carbohydrate

• Fat: 15g

These supper pleasures not only meet your macro diet needs, but they also add a blast of flavor to your evening meal. Feel free to adjust the component amounts to suit your specific nutritional demands and tastes.

Enjoy these filling and nutritious dinners as you end your day on a sweet note.

CHAPTER 4

Snacks and Side Dishes

Satisfy your appetites and maintain your energy levels with these delectable snacks and sides that fit your macro diet goals well. These recipes offer a balance of proteins, carbs, and healthy fats to keep you on track, whether you're searching for a quick snack between meals or a tasty companion to your main courses.

Guacamole with Carrot Sticks

Ingredients:

- 2 ripe avocados, mashed

- 1 small tomato, diced

- 1/4 cup finely chopped red onion

- 1 garlic clove, minced

- fresh lime juice

- salt & pepper to taste

- assorted veggie sticks (carrots, cucumber, bell peppers)

Instructions:

1. Combine mashed avocados, diced tomato, chopped red onion, minced garlic, and lime juice in a mixing dish.

2. Combine until thoroughly blended.

3. Season to taste with salt and pepper.

4. Serve with a variety of vegetable sticks for dipping.

Approximate nutritional value

200 calories

- 3g protein

- 15g carbohydrates

- 15g fat

Greek Yogurt and Berry Parfait

Ingredients:

- 1 cup plain nonfat Greek yogurt

- Strawberries, blueberries, and raspberries

- 1/4 cup granola

- 1 tbsp honey

Instructions:

1. Layer Greek yogurt in a glass or bowl.

2. Cover with a layer of mixed berries.

3. Garnish with granola.

4. Drizzle with honey to finish.

Approximate nutritional value

250 calories

• 20g protein

• 35g carbohydrates

• 5g fat

Platter of Hummus and Veggies

Ingredients:

• Hummus (bought or homemade)

• Assorted vegetable sticks (carrots, celery, cherry tomatoes, and cucumber)

Instructions:

1. Place the hummus in the center of a serving dish.

2. Serve with varied veggie sticks and whole-grain crackers on the side.

3. Serve as a filling and healthful snack.

Approximate nutritional value:

• 300 calories

• 10g protein

• 30g carbohydrates

• 18g fat

Cups of Cottage Cheese and Pineapple

Ingredients:

• 1 cup low-fat cottage cheese

• fresh pineapple pieces

• garnished with mint leaves

Instructions:

1. Layer low-fat cottage cheese and fresh pineapple chunks in individual cups.

2. Garnish with mint leaves if desired.

Approximate nutritional value:

• 220 calories

• 25g protein

• 30g carbohydrates

• 3g fat

Baked Sweet Potato Fries

Ingredients

• Sweet potatoes, sliced into fries

• 1 tablespoon olive oil

• Paprika, garlic powder, and cayenne pepper to taste

Instructions:

1. Preheat the oven to 425 degrees

2. Combine sweet potato fries, olive oil, and seasonings in a mixing bowl

3.Spread out evenly on a baking pan

4. Bake for 20-25 minutes, or until the bacon is crispy

5. Put some salt and pepper on top before you serve.

Approximate nutritional value

180 calories

• 2g protein

• 35g carbohydrates

• 4g fat

Protein-Packed Deviled Eggs

Ingredient

• sliced hard-boiled eggs

• 1/4 cup Greek yogurt

- Dijon mustard

- Seasonings of salt, pepper, and paprika

- Chopped chives for garnish

Instructions:

1. Separate the egg yolks and set them aside in a basin.

2. Whisk together the egg yolks, Greek yogurt, Dijon mustard, salt, pepper, and paprika until smooth.

3. Return the mixture to the egg white halves.

4. Garnish with chives, if desired.

Approximate nutritional value

180 calories

- 15g protein

- 2g carbohydrates

- 12g fat

Nuts and Seeds Trail Mix

Ingredients:

• Dried cranberries

• Almonds

• Walnuts

• Pumpkin seeds

• Sunflower seeds

Instructions:

1. In a mixing dish, combine almonds, walnuts, pumpkin seeds, sunflower seeds, and dried cranberries.

2. Divide into snack-sized portions.

Approximate nutritional value:

• 200 calories

• 8g protein

• 15g carbohydrates

• 15g fat

These snacks and sides are not only tasty but also nutritious, making them ideal additions to your macro diet. You may easily adapt these recipes to fit your preferences and dietary restrictions. Enjoy these delectable snacks guilt-free as you embark on a better lifestyle journey.

CHAPTER 5

Sweet Treats

With these delightful and nutritious sweet snacks, you may satisfy your sweet desire without jeopardizing your macro diet goals. These dishes, which range from guilt-free treats to healthful snacks, strike the perfect mix between fulfilling your appetites and reaching your macro requirements. With these macro-friendly sweet delights, you may discover a world of delectable flavors.

Chocolate Protein Smoothie

Ingredients:

- 1 sprinkling of chocolate protein powder

- 1 banana, frozen

- 1 cup unsweetened almond milk

- 1 tablespoon almond butter

Instructions:

1. Combine chocolate protein powder, frozen banana, almond milk, and almond butter in a blender.

2. For a thicker consistency, add ice cubes.

3. process until a creamy consistency is achieved by blending.

4. Pour into a glass and enjoy this protein-packed chocolate treat.

Approximate nutritional value:

- 300 calories

- 25g protein

- 20g carbohydrates

- 12g fat

Greek Yogurt Parfait with Berries and Granola

Ingredients:

Greek yogurt, berries, and granola

- 1 cup plain nonfat Greek yogurt

- 1/4 cup granola (low-sugar alternative)

- Mixed berries (strawberries, blueberries, raspberries)

- 1 tablespoon honey for drizzling

Instructions:

1. Layer half of the Greek yogurt in a glass or bowl.

2. Sprinkle half of the mixed berries over the yogurt layer.

3. Scatter half of the granola on top of the berries.

4. Continue with the remaining yogurt, berries, and granola.

5. For added sweetness, drizzle honey on top.

Approximate nutritional value:

- 300 calories

- 20g protein

- 40g carbohydrates

- 5g fat

Energy Bites with Banana and Peanut Butter

Ingredients:

- 2 mashed ripe bananas

- 1 cup rolled oats

- 1/4 cup peanut butter

- 1/4 cup honey

- 1/2 cup dark chocolate chips

- 1 teaspoon vanilla essence

- pinch of salt

Instructions:

1. Combine mashed bananas, rolled oats, peanut butter, honey, chocolate chips, vanilla essence, and a bit of salt in a mixing dish.

2. Combine until thoroughly blended.

3. Shape the bits into little balls and lay them on a lined tray.

4. Freeze for 30 minutes before enjoying it.

Approximate nutritional value

180 calories

• 4g protein

• 25g carbohydrates

• 8g fat

Mixed Berry Chia Seed Pudding

Ingredients:

• 2 tbsp chia seeds

• 1 cup unsweetened almond milk

- 1/2 tsp vanilla extract

- mixed berries for topping

- optional: 1 tbsp honey

Instructions:

1. Combine chia seeds, almond milk, and vanilla extract in a jar.

2. Stir well and place in the refrigerator for at least 4 hours, preferably overnight, until the liquid thickens.

3. Before serving, sprinkle with mixed berries.

4. If preferred, drizzle with honey for extra sweetness.

Approximate nutritional value

150 calories

- 4g protein

- 15g carbohydrates

• 8g fat

Apple Baked with Cinnamon and Walnuts

Ingredients:

• 1 cored and sliced apple

• Cinnamon for sprinkling

• 1 tbsp chopped walnuts

• 1 tsp honey (optional)

Instructions:

1. Ensure to preheat the oven to 375 degrees

2. Arrange the apple slices on a baking pan.

3. Garnish with cinnamon and walnuts.

4. Bake for 15-20 minutes, or until the apples are soft.

5. If preferred, drizzle with honey before serving.

Approximate nutritional value:

• Calories: 120;

Protein: 1g;

Carbohydrates: 20g;

Fat: 5g

Protein Ice Cream with Mixed Berries

Ingredients

• 1 cup mixed frozen berries

• 1 scoop vanilla protein powder

• 1/2 cup unsweetened almond milk

Instructions:

1. Combine frozen mixed berries, vanilla protein powder, and almond milk in a blender.

2. Process until a velvety smooth consistency is achieved.

.3. Serve this guilt-free protein-packed ice cream in a bowl.

Approximate nutritional value

200 calories

• 20g protein

• 25g carbohydrates

• 3g fat

Oatmeal Banana Cookies

Ingredients

• 2 mashed ripe bananas

• 1 cup rolled oats

• 1/4 cup raisins or dark chocolate chips

• 1/4 cup chopped nuts (walnuts or almonds)

• 1/2 teaspoon vanilla extract

Instructions:

1. Ensure to preheat the oven to 350 degrees

2. Combine mashed bananas, rolled oats, raisins or chocolate chips, chopped nuts, vanilla essence, and cinnamon in a mixing dish.

3. Place spoonfuls of the mixture on a baking sheet coated with parchment paper

.4.bake until the top turns golden brown, about 15 to 20 minutes.

Approximate nutritional value

160 calories

• 3g protein

• 25g carbohydrates

• 6g fat

These delicious delicacies demonstrate that you can have desserts and snacks while adhering to your macro diet. Whether you want a fruity parfait, a crunchy energy bite, or a creamy protein-packed smoothie, these recipes will satisfy your sweet needs. Enjoy these guilt-free treats as you navigate your way to a healthy and fun macro diet journey.

CHAPTER 6

Eating Out While Following a Macro Diet

1. Maintaining a macro diet does not require you to forego attending social gatherings or giving up eating out if you choose to do so. It is possible to enjoy meals at restaurants while still adhering to your macronutrient goals if you take a strategic approach and are conscious of the nutritional requirements you fulfill. To successfully handle eating out while adhering to a macro diet, the following are some recommendations and principles.

Take a look at the menu online, if it is accessible, before going to a restaurant. This is the first step in the planning process. There are a lot of restaurants that offer nutritional information, which enables you to make more educated choices. When planning your dinner, it is important to take into consideration the different dishes' levels of macronutrients. This preparation helps you avoid making decisions on the spur of the moment and guarantees that you continue to make progress toward your goals.

2. Select Meals Comprised of Protein-Based Options:

Choose meals that are centered around a source of lean protein. All of the following are wonderful options: grilled chicken, fish, lean beef, tofu, or lentils. The consumption of protein is an essential component of a macro diet since it helps to maintain muscular mass and contributes to a feeling of accomplishment. Request that your protein be prepared without the use of excessive oils, sauces, or bread to keep your consumption of carbohydrates and fats under control.

3. Pay Attention to Your Carbohydrate Intake
Pay attention to the amount of carbohydrates you consume, particularly if you are trying to

achieve a particular ratio. Choose options that contain whole grains whenever they are available, such as brown rice, quinoa, or pasta made with whole grains. Avoid consuming an excessive amount of processed carbs, such as white bread or sauces that are high in sugar. You might want to think about replacing typical side dishes with steamed vegetables or a side salad if the restaurant where you are dining offers such options.

4. Pay Attention to Your Fat Intake Even while healthy fats are an important component of your diet, it is still vital to pay attention to the amount of fat you consume, particularly when they are consumed in restaurants. Instead of frying, you should consider using other techniques of cooking such as grilling, baking, or steaming. You will be able to manage the amount of dressings and sauces that you consume if you request that they be served on the side. Choosing foods that contain healthy fats, such as avocados, almonds, or olive oil, can help you improve the nutritional profile of the dish you are preparing.

5. Watch Out for Hidden Calories Meals served at restaurants frequently have hidden calories in the form of extra oils, sauces, and condiments that are not readily apparent. Pose a question to your server about the methods of preparation and the ingredients that were utilized in the dishes. By requesting that dressings, sauces, or butter be given on the side, you will have the ability to limit the amount that is served. Being aware of potential calorie-dense extras that can contribute to exceeding your daily intake is the most important thing concerning this matter.

6. Customization is Absolutely Necessary: Do not be afraid to modify your order to fulfill your own requirements. Dietary preferences and changes are something that the majority of restaurants are ready to accommodate. For instance, you may request a double serving of veggies rather than rice or potatoes, or you could ask for a reduced quantity of a meal that is high in protein if the regular serving is too large.

7. Control the servings: The servings that are served in restaurants are typically larger than the ones that you would cook at home. You might want to think about ordering a to-go box or sharing an entree with a buddy ahead of time so that you can take a portion of your dinner with you. This will not only keep you from overeating, but it will also provide you with a second piece to save for later, which will save you time and work when you are preparing another meal.

8. Give Vegetables Priority: Consume a large quantity of vegetables to increase the volume of your meal and the amount of nutrients you consume without severely affecting your macronutrient targets. Incorporating a wide range of colorful vegetables into your diet, whether it be in the form of a side salad, steaming greens, or a vegetable stir-fry, guarantees that you will provide your body with the necessary vitamins and minerals while also preserving a balanced profile of macronutrients.

9. Maintaining enough hydration is essential since feelings of hunger can sometimes be confused with dehydration. Consume water throughout your meal to maintain proper hydration and to assist in the management of your appetite. Additionally, selecting water as opposed to sugary beverages or alcoholic beverages is a strategic move that contributes to your overall macronutrient strategy.

10. Make Moderation a Practice Although adaptability is necessary, moderation is the most important thing. If you are aware that you will be eating out, you should make adjustments to your other meals during the day. To accommodate the lunch at the restaurant while still remaining within your daily targets, you need to maintain a balance in your consumption of macronutrients throughout the day.

Take, for instance, the situation in which you are dining out: you are at an Italian restaurant. You may choose to consume a chicken breast that has been grilled, accompanied by a side of pasta made with whole grains and a substantial portion of veggies that have been sautéed. Request that the sauce be served on the side so that you may regulate the amount that is served. When it comes to dessert, you might want to think about serving a fruit plate to each other or choosing a small quantity of a dessert that is suitable for your dietary choices.

Consuming food outside of the home while adhering to a macro diet does not have to be difficult. If you prepare ahead, make choices based on accurate information, and exercise moderation, you can enjoy meals in restaurants without compromising your efforts to achieve your intended nutritional goals. Always keep in mind that adaptability is one of the most important aspects of a diet that can be maintained over time, and that finding a balance that is suitable for you is necessary for long-term success. Enjoy your meal!

CHAPTER 7

Troubleshooting and guidance for a successful journey through the macro diet

The decision to embark on a journey of a macro diet is an empowering one; nevertheless, just like any other lifestyle change, it comes with its own set of hurdles. Whether you are experiencing difficulties in adjusting to social circumstances or hitting a plateau, troubleshooting and putting sensible recommendations into action can drastically improve your experience and secure your success over the long term. The following is an all-encompassing handbook that will assist you in resolving typical problems and provide you with helpful advice for navigating your journey through the macro diet.

One of the challenges you face is breaking through a plateau, which is a situation in which your development appears to have stopped.

A word of advice:

plateaus are a typical component of any diet or exercise program. To break through, you should think about modifying the ratios of your macronutrients, increasing the amount of physical activity you do, or integrating periodic refeed days on which you consume slightly more calories to revitalize your metabolism. In addition, you should evaluate whether or not you have been consistent in precisely documenting your food intake; even minor errors might add up over time.

It can be difficult to maintain your macro objectives while attending social gatherings and dining out. This is a challenge for those who are trying to maintain their weight.

A helpful hint is to check out the menus of restaurants online and make choices based on the information you find. Make sure that your friends or relatives who are hosting events are aware of your dietary preferences. When you go to a potluck, bring a meal that is suitable for macronutrients. Not only should you not be afraid to modify your order at restaurants, but you should also be mindful of the quantity proportions.

Concerns Regarding Deficiencies in Nutrients

Confrontation: Worries regarding micronutrient deficits may arise as a result of balancing macronutrients.

As a helpful hint, make sure you are achieving your micronutrient requirements by consuming a wide variety of meals that are rich in nutrients. You should make sure that your diet contains a wide variety of colorful vegetables, fruits, lean proteins, and complete grains. When looking for individualized counsel and direction, you might want to think about consulting a licensed dietitian or a nutritionist.

The Levels of Energy:

The challenge is that you are experiencing low energy levels or feeling exhausted.

It is important to make sure that you are ingesting sufficient calories to meet your energy requirements, particularly if you are active. Additionally, it is essential to drink enough water. If energy levels continue to be a problem, you should reconsider the distribution of your macronutrients and think about modifying the ratios following your activity levels and your own personal preferences.

Turning to food as a means of providing emotional solace is the challenge of emotional eating.

It is a good idea to recognize the emotional triggers that lead to eating and to look for other ways to cope with them, such as keeping a journal, going for a run, or practicing meditation. A supportive environment should be created, and if necessary, a mental health expert should be sought out for guidance. To achieve success over the long run, it is essential to comprehend and deal with emotional eating.

Challenge:

Inaccuracies in tracking macros that lead to departures from your goals. This is the sixth challenge in the macro tracking category.

Advice:

To assure accuracy, make use of trustworthy tracking tools and applications. If at all possible, weigh and measure the stuff you eat. It is especially important to pay attention to portion sizes when dining out. Maintain a consistent schedule of reevaluating and modifying your macro targets on your progress and any changes in your activity levels.

Intake of Fiber:

A Challenge It can be difficult to meet your requirements for fiber intake from your diet.

Tip:

When planning your meals, make sure to include foods that are high in fiber, such as whole grains, legumes, fruits, and vegetables. To avoid discomfort in the digestive tract, gradually increase your consumption of fiber. Because fiber can absorb water, it is important to stay hydrated. Taking a fiber supplement may be necessary, but the consumption of whole foods should take precedence.

Obstacles to Hydration:

Having difficulty keeping up with the necessary amount of hydration level.

You should make it a goal to drink water regularly throughout the day. Keep a water bottle that can be reused on you at all times and set reminders to stay hydrated. For a more flavorful beverage, you might want to think about adding herbal teas or creating a fruit-infused water. Use the color of your urine as a straightforward measure of your level of hydration.

Adaptation to Training:

The challenge of adjusting to changes in your training regimen or increasing activity levels requires you to be flexible.

Your requirements for macronutrients may fluctuate when your level of physical activity changes. Maintain a close eye on your energy levels, make any necessary adjustments to your macronutrient ratios, and make recovery nutrition a top priority after your workout by consuming a healthy mix of carbohydrates and protein. Have patience as your body goes through the process of adapting.

Sustainable Habits:

The challenge consisted of attempting to keep a macro diet that was sustainable over an extended period.

A helpful hint is to concentrate on developing routines that are in line with your preferences and lifestyle. Take advantage of the freedom that comes with your macronutrient targets, and make room for occasional indulgences. The celebration of non-scale triumphs, such as increased levels of energy, improved sleep, and improved performance in the gym, is something to be celebrated. Develop a healthy connection with food by emphasizing enjoying it and maintaining a balance.

Seeking Consultation from Qualified Others

You may be experiencing feelings of being overwhelmed or uncertain about your journey with the macro diet.

You should think about speaking with a licensed dietitian or nutritionist if you are confused about your macronutrient targets, if you have specific health issues, or if you require individualized counsel. Depending on your specific requirements, they can offer individualized guidance and assistance in overcoming any obstacles that may arise.

Consuming food without paying attention to indicators that indicate when you are full or hungry is the challenge of mindful eating.

To practice mindful eating, you should relish each bite, pay attention to cues that indicate when you are hungry and when you are full, and minimize distractions while you are eating. By taking this strategy, one can foster a more positive relationship with food and reduce the likelihood of overeating.

Understanding that the journey of the macro diet is a dynamic process that requires ongoing learning and change is the conclusion. You will be able to improve your experience and develop habits that are sustainable if you adopt these ideas and troubleshoot typical issues. For a successful trip through the macro diet, it is important to keep in mind that flexibility, patience, and self-compassion are essential components.

You should rejoice in your accomplishments, take lessons from your failures, and take pleasure in the uplifting journey toward a lifestyle that is healthier and more balanced.

CHAPTER 8

Sample Meal Plans for a Balanced Macro Diet

A well-organized food plan is essential for a successful macro diet journey. These sample meal plans offer a choice of delicious and nutritious options to suit a variety of dietary preferences and daily calorie requirements. Remember to alter portion sizes based on your unique needs, and if you have special health issues, speak with a healthcare practitioner or certified dietitian.

Meal Plan 1:

Basics in Balance

Adjust portion quantities according to your needs.

Breakfast:

• Scrambled eggs with spinach and tomatoes
• Whole-grain bread

• Slices of fresh orange

Lunch:

• Grilled chicken breast

• Quinoa

• Steamed broccoli and carrots

• Salad of mixed greens with balsamic vinaigrette

Snack:

• Greek yogurt with berries

• A handful of nuts

Dinner:

• Baked salmon

• Asparagus spears

• Quinoa salad with cherry tomatoes and cucumbers

Plant-Based Delights:

Meal Plan 2

Get the recommended amount of protein from plants.

Breakfast:

• Almond milk, banana, and spinach protein smoothie

• Chia seed pudding with mixed berries

Lunch:

• Salad of lentils and chickpeas with mixed greens

• Avocado slices

• Quinoa

Snack:

• Carrot and cucumber sticks with hummus

• Nuts and seeds trail mix

Dinner:

• Stir-fried tofu with broccoli, bell peppers, and snap peas

• Steamed edamame, brown rice

Meal Plan 3:

High-Impact Day

Not suitable for people who need more calories due to increasing physical activity.

Breakfast:

• A protein-rich omelet topped with mushrooms, bell peppers, and feta cheese.

• Avocado on whole-grain bread

Lunch:

- Turkey and veggie wrap on whole-grain tortilla

- Quinoa salad with cherry tomatoes and feta cheese

Snack:

- Cottage cheese with chunks of pineapple

- Oatmeal, peanut butter, and dark chocolate chips energy bits

Dinner:

- Lemon-herb grilled shrimp skewers

- Quinoa

- Roasted sweet potato

- Steamed broccoli and cauliflower

Meal Plan 4:

Simple and Quick Options

Not suitable for anyone with a hectic schedule.

Breakfast:

• Almond milk overnight oats with chia seeds and sliced strawberries

Lunch:

• Cucumber, cherry tomato, and feta cheese chickpea salad

• Pita bread made from whole grains

Snack:

• Almond butter on apple slices

Dinner:

• Chicken stir-fried with assorted vegetables

• Basmati rice

Mediterranean-Inspired Meal Plan 5 Delights

Nota bene: This dish incorporates elements from the Mediterranean diet.

Breakfast:

• Parfait of Greek yogurt, honey, walnuts, and mixed fruit

Lunch:

• Quinoa salad with olives, cherry tomatoes, cucumber, and feta cheese from the Mediterranean

• Chicken breast grilled

Snack:

• Hummus served with whole-grain pita bread

Dinner:

• Lemon-herb baked cod

• Roasted veggies (zucchini, eggplant, bell peppers)

• Couscous with fresh herbs

Meal Plan 6:

Vegetarian Options

Nota bene: A versatile method that combines plant-based and animal-based protein sources.

Breakfast:

• Spinach, banana, protein powder, and almond milk smoothie

Lunch:

• Black bean, corn, avocado, and salsa quinoa bowl• Optional grilled chicken slices

Snack:

• Cottage cheese with bits of mango

• Trail mix

Dinner:

• Tofu stir-fry with broccoli, bell peppers, and snap peas

• Basmati rice

Meal Plan 7:

Low-Carb Alternatives

Note: This is a good option for people who want to limit their carbohydrate intake.

Breakfast:

• A mushroom, spinach, and feta cheese omelet

Lunch:

Grilled fish, cauliflower rice, and steamed asparagus

Snack:

• Salted and peppered avocado slices

• Hard-boiled eggs

Dinner:

• Zucchini noodles with marinara sauce and turkey meatballs

• Mixed green salad with olive oil dressing

Meal Plan 8:

Remixed Comfort Food

Note: These are healthier variations of traditional comfort foods.

Breakfast:

• Banana and oat pancakes

• Honey-sweetened Greek yogurt

Lunch:

• Turkey burger on a whole-grain bun

• Baked sweet potato fries

• Coleslaw with a mild vinaigrette

Snack:

• Baked apple slices topped with cinnamon and granola

Dinner:

• Quinoa-crusted chicken and vegetable skewers

• Roasted Brussels sprouts

Meal Plan 9:

Easy and Healthy

Not suitable for individuals looking for simple solutions.

Breakfast:

• Almond butter on whole-grain bread

• Banana

Lunch:

• Salad with grilled chicken, mixed greens, cherry tomatoes, and vinaigrette dressing

Snack:

- A handful of mixed nuts

- Greek yogurt drizzled with honey

Dinner:

- Lemon-herb baked cod

- Quinoa

- Steamed broccoli

Meal Plan 10:

Protein-Rich Options

Note: Protein-rich alternatives are emphasized for muscle upkeep and satiety.

Breakfast:

- Cottage cheese with peaches

- Scrambled eggs with spinach

Lunch:

• Sweet potato wedges with grilled steak

• Salad of mixed greens with avocado

Snack:

• Almond milk, banana, and protein powder protein smoothie

• Greek yogurt with berries

Dinner:

• Baked rosemary and garlic chicken thighs

• Quinoa

• Roasted Brussels sprouts

CHAPTER 9

Fitness and Macros: A Complete Overview

Integrating activity and a macronutrient-based diet is a great strategy for improving your health, performance, and body composition. Understanding how macronutrients (macros) play an important part in fueling your workouts, promoting recovery, and reaching fitness objectives will help you develop a balanced and sustainable lifestyle. In this comprehensive guide, we'll look at the relationship between fitness and macronutrients, offering recommendations on pre-and post-workout nutrition, macronutrient distribution, and ways to improve your overall fitness journey.

1. The Function of Macros in Fitness:

Macronutrients—proteins, carbs, and fats—are the nutritional building blocks that provide the energy required for physical activity. Each macronutrient performs a specific function:

• Proteins:

Proteins are necessary for muscle repair, growth, and maintenance. Protein consumption is critical for those who engage in weight training or other forms of exercise.

• Carbohydrates:

The primary source of energy for physical exercise. Carbohydrates are stored as glycogen in muscles and play an important function in maintaining energy levels throughout exercises.

• Fats:

Provide a concentrated source of energy and aid in the manufacturing of hormones. It is critical to include healthy fats in your diet for general health and energy balance.

2. Nutrition Before Workout:

Fueling your body before a workout is critical for peak performance. Consider the following pre-workout nutrition guidelines:

• **Timing:**

Eat a healthy meal 2-3 hours before working out, or a smaller snack 30-60 minutes before. This enables for adequate nutritional digestion and absorption.

• **Carbohydrates:**

For rapid energy, choose easily digestible carbs. A banana, whole-grain toast, or a small bowl of muesli are some examples.

• **Proteins:**

A reasonable amount of protein is recommended to help with muscle upkeep. Greek yogurt, a protein shake, or a small bit of lean meat are all good options.

• **Hydration:**

Drink plenty of water before and during your workout. Dehydration can impair performance and recuperation.

3. Nutrition During Exercise:

While intra-workout nutrition isn't always necessary, it can be useful for lengthy or strenuous workouts. Consider the following if your workout lasts longer than an hour:

• Hydration:

Drink water throughout your workout to stay hydrated.

• Carbohydrates:

To maintain energy levels throughout prolonged exercises, include a supply of quickly digestible carbs, such as a sports drink or energy gel.

4. Nutrition Following Exercise:

Optimizing recovery through a post-workout diet is critical for muscle regeneration and glycogen replenishment. Follow these suggestions:

- **Timing:**

Eat a post-exercise meal or snack within 30-60 minutes after finishing your workout to take advantage of your body's increased ability to absorb nutrients.

- **Proteins:**

Make protein a priority to support muscle protein synthesis. Protein shakes, grilled chicken, and Greek yogurt are all options.

- **carbs:**

Complex carbs such as sweet potatoes, brown rice, or whole-grain pasta replenish glycogen stores.

- **Hydration:**

Replace fluids lost during activity by drinking water.

5. Macro Distribution for Fitness Objectives:

The macronutrient distribution in your diet can be modified to certain fitness goals, such as muscle gain, fat loss, or overall health maintenance. Here are some broad suggestions for various fitness goals:

• **Muscle Building (Muscle Hypertrophy):** Increase protein consumption to support muscle growth. Protein intake should range between 1.6 and 2.2 grams per kilogram of body weight. Moderate carbohydrate consumption gives energy for workouts, while healthy fats promote general health.

• **Fat Loss:**

Create a calorie deficit by reducing total calorie consumption while increasing physical activity. Consume enough protein to maintain lean muscular mass. Individual preferences and energy requirements should be considered when adjusting carbohydrates and fats.

- **Maintenance or General Health:**

Maintain a balanced macronutrient distribution. Aim for a modest protein consumption, a well-balanced carbohydrate mix for energy, and healthy fats for overall health.

6. Changing Macros to Account for Activity Levels:

It is critical to tailor your macronutrient intake to your exercise levels to maintain energy and achieve fitness goals. Consider the following modifications:

- **Sedentary Lifestyle:**

If you work at a desk or lead a sedentary lifestyle, alter your carbohydrate consumption to meet your energy demands. To promote general health, prioritize nutrient-dense diets.

- **Moderate exercise:**

Regular physical exercise necessitates a well-balanced macronutrient distribution.

Depending on the intensity and duration of your workouts, adjust your carbohydrate intake.

• Athletes with High Activity Levels: Athletes with hard training programs may require a greater carbohydrate intake to fuel their performance. Make sure you get enough protein for muscle repair and maintenance.

7. Macro Tracking:

Tracking macros entails keeping track of your daily protein, carbohydrate, and fat intake to meet specified nutritional goals. Record and analyze your macronutrient intake using food diaries, mobile applications, or online trackers. Your diet should be adjusted based on your progress, fitness goals, and any changes in activity levels.

8. Customizing Your Approach:

Every person is unique, and there is no one-size-fits-all strategy for exercise and macronutrients. Personal preferences, dietary constraints, and tolerance to specific macronutrient ratios should all be considered. Experiment with several ways until you find a balance that fits your lifestyle and encourages sustainability.

9. Seeking Professional Help:

Consult a certified dietitian or nutritionist if you're unsure how to set your macronutrient targets or if you need personalized assistance. They can make personalized recommendations based on your current health, exercise objectives, and dietary preferences.

10. Maintaining Consistency:

The key to success in any fitness or nutrition quest is consistency. Maintain your macro goals, make adjustments as needed, and celebrate your progress along the way. Long-term well-being is enhanced by developing lasting habits and cultivating a healthy relationship with fitness and nutrition.

Integrating fitness with a macronutrient-based dietary approach enables you to effectively fuel your body, improve performance, and reach your fitness goals. Understanding the importance of macronutrients and using personalized techniques can optimize your fitness journey, whether you're looking to develop muscle, lose weight, or improve your general health. Experiment with various ways, be consistent, and consider obtaining professional advice to fine-tune your nutrition and fitness regimen. Remember that the synergy between fitness and macronutrients is a valuable tool on your journey to a healthier, more active lifestyle.

CHAPTER 10

Tracking Your Fitness Progress: A Comprehensive Guide

Starting a fitness journey entails more than just engaging in physical exercise; it also necessitates a structured approach to tracking and evaluating your progress. Tracking effectively allows you to celebrate accomplishments, discover areas for development, and stay inspired on your journey to health and fitness. In this detailed tutorial, we'll look at numerous ways and essential metrics to help you properly track your development.

1. Set specific objectives:

Setting clear and realistic goals is vital before digging into measuring progress. Having specified, measurable, realistic, relevant, and time-bound (SMART) goals provides a framework for your fitness journey, whether your goals are centered on weight loss, muscle building, enhanced endurance, or improved overall health.

2. Metrics to Monitor Progress:

• Body Dimensions:

• **Waist Circumference:** Measure around your waist at its narrowest point.

• **Hip Circumference:** Measure around the broadest part of your hips.

• **Chest Circumference:** Measure the widest area of your chest.

• **Arm and Leg Circumference:** Measure your upper arm and thigh.

• **Body Mass Index:**

• Get in the habit of regularly weighing yourself, ideally at the same time each day and in the same environment. Remember that swings might occur as a result of factors such as hydration and meal timing. Consider utilizing body weight as one of several measures to get a full picture of your development.

• Percentage of Body Fat:

• While methods for assessing body fat % vary, equipment such as bioelectrical impedance scales, DEXA scans, and skinfold calipers can provide estimations. Monitoring changes in body fat % is frequently more helpful than tracking changes in body weight alone.

• Power and Performance:

• Monitor your strength gains by tracking the weight, repetitions, or length of your exercises. Documenting your performance, whether you're lifting weights, running, or practicing yoga, allows you to track your development and alter your training routine accordingly.

• Cardiovascular Fitness and Endurance:

• Keep track of changes in your capacity to maintain physical activity over time. Improvements in running distance, cycling length, or overall cardiovascular endurance indicate improved fitness levels.

• **Mobility and flexibility:**

• Include flexibility assessments and track your range of motion improvements. Stretching and yoga regularly might help with flexibility and mobility.

• **Eating Habits:**

• Maintain a food journal to keep track of your nutritional intake. This can assist in identifying patterns, assessing adherence to dietary goals, and making informed changes to your nutrition plan.

• **Rest and recuperation:**

• Keep track of your sleep quality, stress levels, and recovery procedures. Adequate rest is essential for general health and can have an impact on your ability to perform and grow in your fitness quest.

3. Methods of Tracking That Are Consistent:

Choose tracking methods that are compatible with your objectives and preferences. Consistency is essential whether you use digital tools, spreadsheets, or handwritten notebooks.

Listed below are a few widely used tracking techniques

• Exercise Apps:

• Use fitness apps to keep track of your exercises, nutrition, and progress images. Apps such as MyFitnessPal, Fitbit, and Strava provide comprehensive capabilities for tracking many parts of your fitness journey.

• Journals on paper:

• Keep a fitness notebook to monitor workouts, objectives, and any changes in measurements or performance. Physical writing can improve mindfulness and commitment.

• Photos of Progress:

• Take images from various angles regularly to visibly document improvements in your physique. These photographs provide as a visual reflection of your progress.

• Measurement Instruments:

• To quantify changes in body composition, use equipment such as body fat calipers, tape measures, or smart scales. For accurate comparisons, use consistent measurement techniques.

4. Frequency of tracking:

The frequency of tracking is determined by user preferences as well as the metrics being tracked.

Consider the following recommendations:

• Weight and Measurements:

Tracking weight and measurements on a weekly or biweekly basis might assist in spotting trends without becoming too focused on day-to-day swings.

• Strength and Performance:

Consistently log your workouts, either after each session or weekly, to measure progress and adapt your training plan as needed.

• Nutrition:

Keep a daily or weekly food record to track your nutritional intake and make informed changes to help you reach your fitness objectives.

• Overall Progress Review:

Schedule full monthly or bi-monthly assessments of all metrics to analyze the big picture of your fitness journey.

5. Changing Your Approach:

Reevaluate your goals and tracking systems regularly. If you routinely fulfill your goals, consider pushing yourself even higher. If your progress is stalled, consider nutrition, exercise intensity, or recovery tactics. Based on your findings, modify your approach.

6. Non-Scale Victories Should Be Celebrated:

Changes in body weight do not define progress. Non-scale triumphs, like increased strength, endurance, flexibility, or commitment to a healthy lifestyle, should be celebrated. These triumphs have a big impact on your general well-being.

7. Be Wary of Plateaus:

Any fitness journey is certain to encounter plateaus. Plateaus may not always mean failure, but they may suggest the need for modifications. To overcome plateaus, reassess your goals, change your workout program, or seek advice from fitness professionals.

8. Pay Attention to Your Body:

Take note of how your body feels and reacts to your physical program. Consider modifying your workout intensity or including extra rest days if you feel chronic fatigue, soreness, or indicators of overtraining. Rest and recovery are essential for long-term fitness achievement.

9. Professionals should be consulted:

Consider speaking with fitness specialists, dietitians, or healthcare doctors if you are having difficulty tracking your progress. They can offer specialized advice, solve concerns, and provide guidance to help you improve your fitness journey.

10. Maintain a Positive Attitude and Be Patient:

Fitness is a lifelong endeavor, and progress is not necessarily linear. Maintain an optimistic attitude, be patient, and recognize that lasting changes take time. Concentrate on the good improvements you've implemented and the overall improvement in your health.

Recording your fitness development effectively requires a combination of quantitative measurements, consistent recording methods, and a thoughtful attitude toward your general well-being. You'll acquire vital insights into your progress by defining clear goals, using various tracking tools, and celebrating both scale and non-scale wins. Remember that everyone's fitness path is different, and changes should be made based on personal preferences and input from your body. Accept the process, stay consistent, and revel in the ongoing improvement of your health and fitness.

CONCLUSION

In conclusion, going on a fitness journey is a transforming experience that goes beyond physical activities. A holistic approach that includes clear goal-setting, constant tracking, and an unrelenting dedication to well-being is the key to success. Individuals may create a sustainable lifestyle that promotes holistic health by recognizing the synergistic relationship between fitness and diet.

Setting goals that are specific, measurable, achievable, relevant, and time-bound (SMART) creates a road map for achievement. A well-defined target gives the required direction for one's fitness journey, whether the goal is muscle building, weight loss, or improved general health.

Tracking progress is an important part of the process since it provides physical evidence of hard effort and dedication. A thorough assessment of one's evolution can be obtained by using a range of indicators, ranging from body measurements and weight to strength and performance benchmarks. Consistency is essential, whether through digital apps, handwritten journals, or progress images, to ensure a consistent and continuous record of accomplishments and places for growth.

Understanding the significance of macronutrients in fueling workouts and supporting recuperation improves the fitness journey even further. Integrating proteins, carbs, and fats in a balanced way helps with energy demands, muscle maintenance, and overall health. An optimized nutrition plan includes personalizing macronutrient ratios depending on specific fitness objectives and activity levels.

The capacity to change tactics is critical along this journey. Recognizing plateaus as chances for refinement rather than setbacks enables for continuing advancement. Celebrating both scale and non-weight wins, such as increased strength, endurance, and commitment to a healthy lifestyle, reinforces fitness's favorable impact on overall well-being.

Listening to the body and making conscious changes to workout intensity, recuperation tactics, and nutritional choices promotes a long-term and healthy connection with fitness. Seeking expert advice when necessary ensures a well-informed and balanced approach to health.

Finally, the result of these efforts is a dynamic, lifelong path toward well-being. Every person's journey is distinct, formed by own tastes, struggles, and accomplishments. The commitment to positive transformation, patience, and an appreciation for the continual growth of one's health and fitness are the threads that run through this journey. Embracing the process, remaining positive, and celebrating tiny accomplishments transform the fitness journey into a joyful and meaningful way of life.

www.ingramcontent.com/pod-product-compliance
Lightning Source LLC
Chambersburg PA
CBHW070852260726
48661CB00004B/1362